HOMOEOPATHY
MADE HANDY

DR. KAILSH PRASAD

This book is dedicated to my beloved teacher, Sri. P.R. Sarkar, without his grace and constant motivation this could not have become possible.

"The object of the art of healing is to cure a patient, both physically and mentally. So the main question is not to uphold any particular school of medical science; rather, the key task is the welfare of the patient."

Prabhat Ranjan Sarkar

CONTENTS

AUTHOR'S NOTE

I am only a humble student in this vast branch of medicine. I have tried my best to keep this book as precise and simple that even a novice to this science can understand and apply the remedies on his own and can benefit not only himself but also his dear and near ones.

If my little contribution can help remove the suffering of even a few, I will consider my labour rewarded.

<u>INTRODUCTION TO HOMOEOPATHY</u>

The word "Homoeopathy" is derived from the Greek word which means similarity of symptoms. As the name suggests it is based on the doctrine of **like cures like**, according to which if a substance which causes the symptoms of a disease in a healthy person will cure similar symptoms in sick person. Thus by overlapping the symptoms we can cure a disease. For example an onion is a substance that makes your eyes water and nose burn. So if you are having hay fever with watering eye and burning nose, a few doses of Homoeopathic onion (Allium. Cepa.) can relieve it.

BENEFITS OF HOMOEOPATHY

- ➢ Homoeopathic remedies are extremely safe and free of side effects.

- ➢ Like antibiotics, homoeopathic remedies do not kill the germs or virus directly, but rather, stimulate the immune system to do the healing. So germs can never develop a resistance to Homoeopathic remedies, in other words where antibiotic fails homoeopathy works.

- ➢ Homoeopathic remedy removes the toxins from the body whereas conventional drugs increase the toxins.

- ➢ People who are allergic to antibiotics or other drugs can use Homoeopathic remedies.

ADMINISTER OF REMEDY

Generally two remedies are shown in bracket and should be given in alternation. Alternation means one remedy after the other in an interval of at least two hours. If relief occurs decrease the dose and stop. If no relief is obtained after three doses of each remedy, change to other combination, if there is one. For example (Belladona, Chamomilla), it indicates a combination that means first Belladona-30 should be taken then after an interval of two hours Chamomilla-30 should be taken and continue the same until one gets relief, or switch to other combination if mentioned.

For single remedy mentioned, they can be taken in morning, noon and evening three times a day. Results should be available in maximum of three days otherwise stop. If it shows any relief, first decrease and then stop.

Never go on giving medicines indefinitely.

SUGGESTED REMEDIES AND ITS POTENCY

(Remedies not shown with potency are of 30th potency otherwise it is mentioned)

The remedies listed here are those that are mentioned throughout this book. These are the remedies which are most commonly used in acute situations and should occupy the position in home kit.

Most of the remedies indicated here are the polycrest remedies, remedies that respond to a wide range of symptoms and are of varied uses.

List of suggested remedies :

A

1. Abrotanum. (Abrot.)

2. Aciditum sulphur. (Acid-sulp.)

3. Aconitum napellus. (Acon.)

4. Allium cepa. (All-c.)

5. Ammonium carbonicum. (Am-c.)

6. Anacardium orie. (Anac-ori.)

7. Antimonium crudum. (Ant-c.)

8. Apis mellifica. (Apis.)

9. Argentum nitricum. (Arg-n.)

10. Arnica montana. (Arn.)

11. Arsenicum album. (Ars.)

B

1. Bacillinum. (Bacill.)

2. Baryta carbonica. (Bar-c.)

3. Baryta muriatica. (Bar-m.)

4. Belladonna. (Bell.)

5. Bellis perennis. (Bell-p.)

6. Berbaris aquifolium. (Berb-aqui.)

7. Borax. (Bor.)

8. Bryonia. (Bry.)

9. Bismuth metalicum (Bismuth-met.)

C

1. Cactus grandiflorus. (Cact.)

2. Calcarea carbonica. (Calc-c.)

3. Calcarea fluorica. (Calc-f.)

4. Calcarea iodate. (Calc-i.)

5. Calcarea phosphorica. (Calc-p.)

6. Colophylum thalic. (Colo-tha.)

7. Cantharis. (Canth.)

8. Carbo vegetabilis. (Carb-v.)

9. Causticum. (Caust.)

10. Chamomilla. (Cham.)

11. China off. (Chin.)

12. Cimicifuga. (Cimic.)

13. Cina. (Cina.)

14. Colocynthis. (Coloc.)

15. Conium. (Con.)

16. Crataegus. (Crataeg.)

17. Cuprum metallicum. (Cupr-met.)

D

1. Digitalis. (Dig.)

2. Dioscorea. (Dios.)

3. Drosera. (Dros.)

E

1. Eupatorium purfolitum. (Eup-pur.)

2. Euphrasia. (Euphr.)

F

1. Flouric acid. (Fl-ac.)

G

1. Gelsemium. (Gels.)

2. Glonoine (Glon.)

3. Graphites. (Graph.)

H

1. Hepar sulphuris. (Hep.)

2. Hyoscyamus. (Hyos.)

3. Hypericum. (Hyper.)

I

1. Ignatia. (Ig.)

2. Iodum. (Iod)

3. Ipecacuanha. (Ip.)

4. Iris versicolor. (Iris-v.)

K

1. Kali bichromicum.(Kali-b.)

2. Kali bromatum. (Kali-br)

4. Kali Iodium. (Kali-iod.)

5. Kali muriaticum. (Kali-m)

L

1. Lac defloratum. (Lac-def)

2. Lobelia inflata. (lob-inf.)

3. Lycopodium. (Lyco.)

M

1. Magnesia phosphorica. (Mag-p.)

2. Mercurius corrosivus. (Merc-c.)

3. Mercurius vivus or sol. (Merc-s.)

4. Myristica.

N

1. Natrum muriaticum. (Nat-m.)

2. Natrum phosphoricum. (Nat-p.)

3.Natrum sulphuricum. (Nat-s.)

4.Nitric acid. (Nit-ac.)

5.Nux vomica. (Nux-v.)

P

1.Paeonia. (Paen.)

2.Phytolacca. (Phyt.)

3.Podophyllum. (Podo.)

4.Pulsatilla. (Puls.)

R

1. Ratanhia. (Rat.)

2.Rhus toxicodendro. (Rhus-t.)

3.Ruta graveolens. (Ruta.)

S

1. Sabal Serrulata. (Sabal.)

2. Sabina (Sabin.)

3. Sanguinaria. (Sang.)

4. Sepia. (Sep.)

5. Silicea. (Sil.)

6. Spongia tosta. (Spong.)

7. Staphysagria. (Staphy.)

8. Sulphur. (Sulph.)

9. Symphytum. (Symph.)

10. Syzgium jambolanum. (Syz.)

T

1. Thuja. (Thuj.)

2. Trillium cernum. (Tril-c.)

U

1. Uranium nitricum. (Uran.)

2. Ustilago maydis. (Ust.)

V

1. Veratrum virioe. (Verat-v.)

2. Viburnun opulus. (Vib-o.)

EMERGENCIES

CONDITIONS : REMEDIES

1. Any injury : Arnica (two hourly)

2. Before and after tooth extraction : (Arnica, Hypericum-200)

3. Fracture pains before bone is set right : Arnica (two hourly)

4. For quick union of bones : Symphy. (three doses a day for one week)

5. Sprains : (Arnica, RhusTox)

6. Crushed fingers : Hypericum-1M (three doses only)

7. Stretching pain after operation : Staphy.

8. Gas in abdomen after operation : (Carbo Veg, China)

9. Acute Asthma : (Aconite,Arnica,Ipecac) or (Arsenic, Nat Sulph)

10. Acute colic : (Colocynth 3X, Mag Phos-1M) or (Colocynth 3X, Dioscoria 6)

11. Gall stone colic : (Bellodonna, Calc.carb)

12. Kidney stone pain : (Berberis V.Q, Belladonna)

13. Hangover (alcohol) : Nux.Vom.

14. Acute Dysentery: (Colocynth 3X, Merc. Cor.)

15. Vomits with colic : Bismuth

16. Diarrhoea : (Podophylum,China)

17. Hiccough after operation : Hyoscyamus

18. Cuts and wounds : Hypericum-1M and Hypericum Q.(should be applied externally)

19. Pain in eye after operation : Rhus Tox (four doses only)

20. Burns: Cantharis 200 (two hourly , four doses only)

21. Acute gas formation: (Carbo Veg, China)

22. Collapse: (Arsenic,Carbo Veg, China)

23. Vomit and Diarrhea at a time: (Arsenic, China, Veratrum Alb.)

24. Continued Nausea: Ipecac

25. Heart problems (we can get time to reach a doctor) : Aconite and Arnica (at same time,every half an hour) or Cactus-6 (four doses)

26. Pulse sinking (goes beyond feeling):* Digitalis (three doses only)

*Digitalis is inimical with China

27. Eye Inflammation with water and pus discharge: Euphrasia or Argent. Nit. or Mere.Cor.

PROBLEMS OF CHILDHOOD

ALIMENTS : REMEDIES

1. Fever : (Belladonna, Chamomilla)

2. Diarrhoea : (Chamomilla, Podophyllum)

3. Cramps : (Belladonna, Chamomilla)

4. Cough Teasing : (Belladona, Chamomilla)

5. Whooping cough : (Bryonia, Ipecac)

6. Measles : (Aconite, Pulsatilla) or (Arsenic, Rhus Tox)

7. Mumps : (Phytolacca, RhusTox)

8. Tonsilitis : (Baryta Mur) or (Belladonna, Hepar Sulph)

9. Dwarfish : BarytaCarb-200 (twice a week) and Sulphur-30 (once a week)

10. Chest affections : (Aconite,Bryonia) and Sulphur (one dose only)

11. Worms : (Cina-30, Natrum Phos 3X)

12. Headache : (Nat Mur, Calc Phos)

13 .Masturbation habit : Staphysagaria

14. Thin neck : Nat Mur

15. Weak bones : Calc.Carb-1M (one dose only)

16. Glands enlarged : Iodium

17. Marasmum with thin legs : Abrotanum

18. Appetite absent : (Thuja, RhusTox)

PROBLEM OF LADIES

1. Leucorrhoea: (Nat.Sulph.,Mag.Phos.) or (Pulsatilla, Caulophylum)

2. Menses relating to :

- Profuse: (Ustilago,Trillium Q) and Calc.Iod.(Once a week for four weeks)
- Scanty: (Pulsatilla, Nat.Mur.)
- Irregular: Nat.Mur.(one dose in morning) and Sepia(one dose in evening, both once a week)
- Painful: Mag Phos-1M (one dose a day, twice a week), Colocynth (three hourly when pains)

3. Frequent urination in newly married : Staphysagaria

4.Pregnancy:

- Nausea during pregnancy : Ipecac
- Legs heavy & aching : Bellis
- Abdomen pain: Viburnum Op. Q or (Cimicifuga, Mag.Phos.)
- False pain: Caulophylum

- Abortion threatened: (Viburnum Op Q, Cimicifuga) or Sabina (two doses only)
- After delivery (to prevent infection) : Arnica (four doses a day,in an interval of two hours, for two days only)
- Milk breast (breast sore, hard & fever): (Bryonia, Phytolacca)

5. No milk in breast : Lac. Defloratum (four doses a day for two days only)

5. Menopause :

- Headache and hot flushes: Sanguinaria (four doses only) or Belladonna, Glonoine & Chamomilla(two days only)
- Back pains : Rhus.Tox.

HEAD

1. Bald : For first two days Floric acid and Silicea alternately, then after two weeks Bacillinum-200 weekly for four weeks.

2. Dandruff: Arsenic, Nat. Sulph.,Thuja-6 (three days only)

3. Migraine:-

- due to acidity : (Iris. V. , Nux.V.)
- due to meno-problems : Sanguinaria(three times a day)
- due to anemia : (Calc. Phos., Nat. Mur.)

EYE

1. Inflammation : Euprasia

2. Styes : (Pulsatilla, Silicea) or staphysagria

3. Strain : (Calc.Phos., Ruta)

NOSE

1. Common Cold : (Aconite,Pulsatilla) or (Arsenic, Nat. Sulph.) or (Dulcamarh, Nat.Sulph.)

2. Sinus : (Puls, Kali.Bich) or (Rhus.Tox., Phytolacca)

3.Nose Block : (Carbo.Veg., Lycopodium, Nux.Vom)

THROAT

1.Hoarse voice : Carbo.Veg. and Causticum (two days only)

2. Swollen,infected & burning: (Kali.Iod. , Phytolacca)

SKIN

1. Acne : Kali Brom-30 (once every week) and Berberis Aqui. Q (five drops with water twice daily)

2. Warts : Causticum and Staphysagria (two days and repeat after two weeks)

3. Urticaria : (Apis-1M, Nat.Mur-1M) or (Hepar Sulph, Arsenic,Rhus.Tox.)
(two days only)

4. Itches : (Lobelia In., Rhus.Tox)

5. Itches with postules : (Rhus. Tox., Croton)

6. Corns on soles : Antim Cruel (three doses once a week)

7. Whitlow (painful boil at the end of finger): Myristica(two hourly)

MOUTH

1. Apthae(ulcers or blisters): Borax (3 doses for two days only) or (Nitric Acid , Natrum Sulph, Arsenic)

2. Bleeding gums : (CarboVeg., Silicea) or (Kali.Iod., Hepar Sulph)

EAR

1. Pain : (Pulsatilla, Chamomilla)

2. Pus discharge : (Kali. Mur., Pulsatilla) or (Mezerium, Merc Sol.)

3. Wax Excess : Conium (two doses only)

LIPS

1.Crack : (Nat. Mur., Rus Tox.)

2.Corners Crack : Antim. Cond.(three doses for two days and repeat after two weeks)

NECK

1. Cervical spondylosis : (Colocynth, Rhus.Tox., Arsenic)

2. Stiffneck : (Colocynth, Rhus.Tox., Arsenic)

CHEST

1. Cough :
(Bryonia,Ipecac)or(Aconite,Spongia) or (Bryonia, Ammon.Carb.)

2. Pleurisy : (Aconite, Bryonia, Sulphur)

STOMACH & INTESTINE

1. Acidity : (Pulsatilla, Acid Sulph.)

2. Gastric/Indigestion: (Carbo.Veg.,China)

3. Dysentery: (Colocynth 3X,Merc. Cor)

4. Loose motion due to ice cream, unsuitable fruits etc. : (Carbo.Veg., Arsenic) or (China, Nat.Sulph)

URINARY TROUBLE

1. Sugar in blood & urine: (Syzy Q,Uran.Nit.)

2. Burning sensation while urination: Cantharis 200 (two doses only)

3. Enlarged Prostrate : (Sabal Serul Q, Calc. Fluor)

SEX PROBLEMS

1. Impotency : Lycopodium CM (one dose only) then on next day Carbo.Veg.-200 (one dose a month for three months only)

2. Other related problem : Staphysagria
(two doses once a week for four weeks)

FEVER

1. Flu : (Bryonia, Nux.Vom.) or (Baptisia,
Gelsemium)

2. Continued fever : (Bryonia,Rhus.Tox.)

3. Continued fever with throat infection :
(Rhus.Tox.,Phytolacca)

4. Intermittent : RhusTox & Arsenic (when
in fever), then Sulphur, China & Arsenic
(when no fever)

5. Intermittent (much aching) :
Rhus.Tox.(when in fever), Eupat.Perf.& Nat.
Mur. (when no fever)

6. Sudden high fever with bursting
headache : (Belladona, Chamomilla)

7. Sudden high fever with thirst,restlessness
due to dry cold wind: Aconite (three doses
only) and Sulphur (one dose only on the
next day)

ANUS

1.Piles : (Sulph, Nux.Vom.) or (Ratanhia 6, Peonia 6)

2.Fissure : Flourine Acid and Silicea (two days and repeat after a week for a month)

3.Prolapsus (rectum) : (Ruta, Calc.Phos.)

FITS

1. Epilepsy : Cuprum Met. 30 and Calc.Carb.-1M (one dose from each and repeat after one month)

2. Hysteria : Ignatia and Nat Mur(once a week for four weeks only)

DEBILITY

1. General weakness : (Carbo.Veg., China)

2. Weakness after drains: (Carbo.Veg., China)

BLOOD PRESSURE (RELIEF ONLY)

1. High : (Belladona, Glonoine)

2. Low : Crataegus Q (two dose only)

PAINS

1. Knee pain : Rhus.Tox, Ruta & Calc.Phos. (one week only)

2. Back pain : Pulsatilla & RhusTox (three days only)

3. Sciatica : Colocynth, RhusTox, Arsenic (one week only)

BITES

1. Mosquito bites : Cantharis 200 (two doses only)

2. Bug/Insect bites : Hypericum or Arsenic. or Ledum P.

3. Bee sting : Urtica Urens (apply internally as well as externally)

MENTAL ILLNESS AND PHOBIA

1. Examination phobia in students:

- Fright of examination : Anacardium Orie.
- Terror of anticipation : Argentum Nit.
- Over nervousness in exams : Sil.
- Depression about passing exams : Lycopodium

2. Fear of loanliness : Sep.

3. Fear of darkness, thunder storm : Phos.

4. Enormous grief due to accident, death of loved ones etc, : Ignatia

5. Sleeplessness : Kali. Phos.

6. Weak memory : Anacardium Ori. (twice a week one month only)

Do all the good you can,

By all the means you can,

In all the places you can,

At all the times you can,

To all the people you can,

As long as ever you can.

DR. KAILASH PRASAD

www.ingramcontent.com/pod-product-compliance
Lightning Source LLC
Chambersburg PA
CBHW060344290526
45791CB00004B/1528